HEALTH IN POETRY

Peta Zafir

Health in Poetry

Book 2

©2021 Peta Zafir

All rights reserved.

No part of this book may be reproduced in any form or by any electronic or mechanical means, including information storage and retrieval systems, without written permission from the author, except in the case of a reviewer, who may quote brief passages embodied in critical articles or in a review.

Trademarked names appear throughout this book. Rather than use a trademark symbol with every occurrence of a trademarked name, names are used in an editorial fashion, with no intention of infringement of the respective owner's trademark.

The information in this book is distributed on an "as is" basis, without warranty. Although every precaution has been taken in the preparation of this work, neither the author nor the publisher shall have any liability to any person or entity with respect to any loss or damage caused or alleged to be caused directly or indirectly by the information contained in this book.

Peta Zafir Publishing
www.petazafir.com

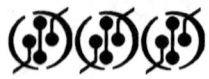

ISBN 978-0-6452140-2-4

Peta Zafir Publishing
www.petazafir.com
Peta Zafir You Tube Channel

BOOKS BY PETA ZAFIR
Health in Poetry Book 1
Health in Poetry Book 2
Book of Sayings Book 1
Book of Sayings Book 2
Book of Sayings Book 3
Book of Sayings Book 4
Scenar For Beginners

All books are available in print and eBook format from:
www.petazafir.com/books

Dedication

I dedicate this book to the toxic people who were brought into my life enabling me to learn many universal lessons. These people are no longer in my life, yet they taught me to care for myself, make myself a priority and understand that I need to make decisions to create my peace and contentment.

Many times, we try to repair, put up with, excuse and tolerate people who bring unhappiness and emotional pain to us. This is due to Fear and Conditioning. These people are learnings for us, forcing us to develop the strength to say NO.

NO, you cannot do this to me. NO, I do not have to act that way. NO, I am entitled to have a calm and loving life, determined by my own needs.

Today my inner voice says that I only have people in my life who are Unconditionally Loving, Supportive and Loyal.

I wish to thank you for coming into my life and bringing me these very hard and sad lessons; yet out of trauma and collapse, I received the gift of understanding and growth.

I have so much serenity and happiness now and wonderful strong healthy boundaries because you were in my life and I let you go.

Thank you to the toxic people who taught me that I am important, such a necessary important lesson.

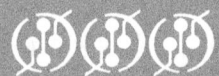

The world is full of beautiful things
People who care and the joys that they bring
Skies that are blue and seas deep and clear
Mountains and valleys and open frontiers
Our Food and our water are needed for health
We cannot go forward focused only on wealth
Businesses must not release all of their waste
They need to be mindful, not develop in haste
We need to unite and stop the destruction
We need to take action and slow down production
We inhabit this earth for a limited time
Make sure when you leave you have not caused decline.

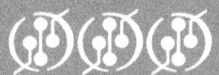

A new day is starting, the time is now here
Time passes swiftly right through the whole year
Our work increases, our holidays pass
Travels exciting, yet home is what lasts
Remember when travelling to places unknown
Take supplements, herbs and oils that you own
Your health is important, so don't take a risk
Support your immunity and make a health list
Get others to help and direct you with this
And live your life fully, in healthy strong bliss.

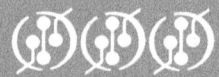

Learning is a part of Life
And though we live through joy and strife
It is the way we battle through
And the people who stay next to you
Our paths can sometimes seem so clear
And we may have ones close and dear
Yet from the side comes lessons to learn
And it is this that creates concern
However, do not ponder the problems long
Work through the issues, stay focused and strong
Don't live your life with sadness and fear
Work hard to make your pathway Clear.

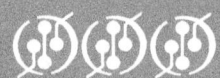

Every day is a brand new start
Allowing you to open your heart
Think of the life that you want to do
Think of the actions that you wish to include
Connect with the people that make you feel grand
Reach out and ask for a kind helping hand
Make this year, a year of great Joy
Set out a strategy and commence to deploy
Get up and complete just one thing today
Do it the best that you can in your way
Don't compare to another, don't care what is said
You have your gifts, find your path, and then move ahead.

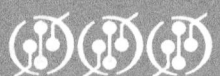

This Day it brings a life renewed
Morning is here and a happy mood
The trees are green and the birds are singing
Perfumes released and flowers are blooming
This is a time of repair and rebirth
As nature opens and sprouts from the earth
Unfortunately for some this is not a good time
It brings great discomfort with allergy signs
Coughs and sneezes, runny noses too
Very unpleasant for more than a few
Keep moving forward and look for a way
To get your immunity stronger today.

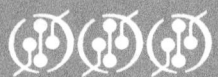

Travel the world and then come back
Learn new skills and extend your track
Vary your workplaces and studies too
All of this knowledge will nourish you
There is much to achieve in your journey through life
We have Paths and choices to avoid all the strife
And sometimes these works and at other times No
So remember stand tall and make your life Go.

The end of the year is coming fast
We celebrate workers from now and the past
Their strength and their energy, up to today
As a nation we need to praise them everyway
So strong and healthy we all must be
To play with our families and swim in the sea
Work hard through the week and visit with friends
And clear past emotions and help yourself mend.

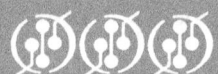

The months they go and the years pass by
Time moves so swiftly in the blink of an eye
Make time for the people who are important to you
Don't let space and work divide loved ones in two
Life goes so quickly and people move on
And don't let them go without singing their song
So spend your time fully don't worry about strife
Make people important and priorities in life
Don't stay in sadness, or isolate in your shell
Force yourself out and connect and be well
We're not meant to live, shut away and alone
Join your community, pick up the phone.

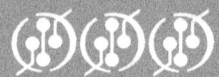

Disease and sickness is all around
And so many treatments are to be found
What one to choose, and which one will work
Will it make you better or could it hurt
It's important to see a person you trust
Talk with them, question them, this is a must
Never just follow what others may say
Connect with your body it'll show you the way
The body can make a strong healthy healing
However, you need to trust how you are feeling
Great health comes from the food that we eat
Great health comes from the emotions we meet
Great health comes from the choices we make
So make them today and start to feel great.

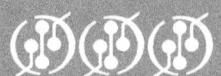

October sees the clock rewind
As Queensland will be left behind
As Daylight saving starts to go
And business' then will lose its flow
However, keep your body strong
Support your health and don't do wrong
Clean up your foods, get sugar out
And if you smoke then have no doubt
That if you don't throw them away
Your healthy body will just decay
So start your plan and do it now
And talk with others they'll show you how.

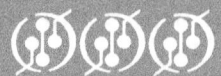

The end of the year has come so fast
The months have vanished, the year's flown past
The sun is shining, the cold has gone
The beach is beckoning, and birds sing their song
Take time to connect with Land and Sea
Take time to focus on what you need
Now is the time, focus on yourself
Now is the time, focus on your Health
So don't wait a second, or say maybe one day
Now is the time, health is not far away.

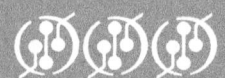

Hello to Summer, you are here
Indicating it's nearly the end of the year
The nights are humid, the days so hot
We need to consider what foods to allot
Waters is first and needs to be pure
Add ¼ of a lemon, to make it the cure
You need to be moving and walking's a must
Fresh fruits & green drinks are something to trust
The sun is so healthy, toxin free food is too
Remember to ground, walk the beach without shoes
Summer flu can be present, don't let it within
Build a strong immune system and let happiness in.

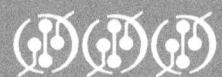

Yet another month is next in line
We're looking at changes in health as a sign
The smallest twinge, a minute ache
Are indicators that there are changes to make
Listen to your body, hear how it flows
The warnings are clear and the processes slow
Take action immediately, don't wait a day
Change what you're doing and it may go away
The body repairs, don't hesitate
If left unattended, may accelerate
Work on clearing the pain and the blocks
By calming and balancing your circadian clock.

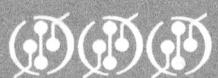

The months are all passing and oh what a year
Ups and downs and lifetime fears
Sickness, pain and sadness too
Felt by all yet some work through
The mental stress of life is high
And not all of us can sail right by
We need to stop and face the woes
Before we learn to let them go
Take action now and do the work
Don't let these growing feelings lurk
Find people who will support you now
That some action and find out how.

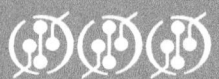

We've now reached the end of a turbulent year
Had ups and downs, feeling joys and fear
And as we live through the upheavals in life
Our lessons are taught, as we sift out the strife
Everything that has happened to you in your past
Work on them, clear them out, start to move fast
Every fresh day is the start of the new
Get up and make choices, direct your life too
When your awake think of health and good food
Then through the day stay in touch with your mood
Never let anyone heavy your load
Find your life's Light and follow that road.

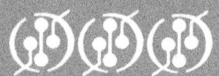

The year now quickly speeds to the end
And we remember the things we tried to amend
The family we spoke with, the friends that we made
The people we meet and the places we stayed
There are so many things that in hindsight we'd change
There are things we'd do differently, life rearranged
Never look backwards it achieves no result
They're the choices we made and the lessons we got
Have a wonderful Day, relax and have fun
Laugh often, stay healthy and sit in the sun
Eat wisely, drink carefully and focus on you
And start everyday completely renewed.

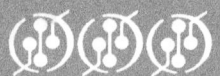

The end of year is approaching fast
Jobs to do and the weeks they pass
Make sure the buying of presents you get
Doesn't deplete your monetary net
Keep to a budget and take your time
Leave credit cards home & finances in line
The holiday season is family and friends
These are important and you can depend
Lift your spirit and start to soar
Celebrate life as it changes once more
Give thanks to all you have known and seen
Bring laughter and joy and much holiday glee.

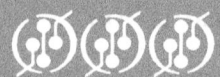

Here we are at the end of the Year
Holidays coming and Christmas Cheer
Loved ones together and lots of Fun
Swimming and basking in Surf and Sun
Make sure that you eat 95% good
The other 5% may be not what you should
However, it is, a time of rejoice
A Time to be merry and sing at top voice
Keep yourself safe with great Joy and good Health
And see in the New Year helping Body and Self.

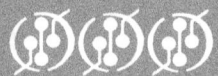

There are things that happen that are unplanned
And wrongs that you will experience firsthand
There will come a time in your life to review
To take stock of the part which you added too
We can always find fault and blame another
We can say it's maybe your father or mother
However, when you need your life to change
It's your thoughts that will need to be rearranged
You need to understand the input and strife
You need to look deeper at your part in life
Work through the past and slowly let go
Then open your life to the path where you glow.

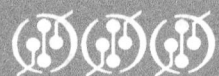

The holidays are so very near
And this can cause some inward fear
Family coming or staying away
Mixing with children or alone on the day
Loneliness is prevalent now
So try to reach out to another somehow
Whether a visit or call on a phone
Check to make sure others aren't left alone
Always stay focused on you and your health
And be extra careful not to spend all your wealth
Make sure that you walk, eat well and stay bright
And welcome each new day with strength & foresight.

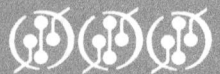

Every year the New Year starts
Suggesting the year, it will Be
With lots of activities and actions for all
And treatments just solely for Me
Munching through Christmas
Celebrating New Year
The holiday season has passed
Now back to the routine
Of work, friends and Fun
Making sure that your Health is to Last.

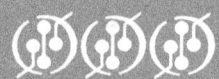

Christmas has passed and New Year too
The next year now is open to you
We've all eaten sugars, the cakes and the treats
The pies and the ice-cream and all of the sweets
We connected with loved ones, had a great break away
Now we'll reset our bodies in a clean healthy way
You can make a new future and see where it leads
You can choose a new pathway with healthy new deeds
Whatever you've done over holiday time
Today is the time to get back into line.

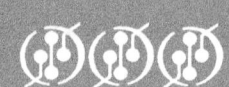

We're off and starting another Year
Each year arrives with abundant cheer
The holidays past, New Year has gone
The indulgences finished and fun carriers on
Try to be healthy and keep living strong
Hopefully nothing for you has gone wrong
Look forward to seeing what happens this year
Start new adventures without holding Fear
Think of your dreams and focus anew
Ready to conquer all obstacles too.

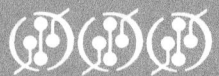

Hurray Hurray we made it through
Another year has commenced for you
This is the time for planning your path
Making your goals, and having a laugh
Working towards a happy fun end
Adding a drop of contentment then blend
Workplace and family need to be strong
And focus on health, must be all lifelong
Start the year off with acceptance of you
Filter the people that you will let through.

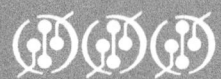

Here we are a brand new year
I hope you had some New Year cheer
Now back we go to work again
And get into balance and maintain
Have you indulged in lots of sweets
Biscuits, lollies and yummy treats
Now is the time, no more sugar lust
Clean healthy living is surely a must
Make healthy choices that is the way
Focus on you all through the day.

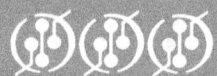

The year's taken off and February's here
And the focus now goes onto those you hold Dear
On the 14th we celebrate Valentine's Day
Share a gift and a thought, or a Health resort stay
Give them an hour to relax and slow down
Replenish their energy, with no one around
Feet to be massaged, a Facial is done
Wrapped in a Blanket, they're your number one
I know that you value them all the year through
But Valentine's Day is a special day too.

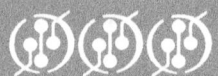

All the months they come and go
Now April has begun to flow
With April fool's day be aware
Drink water is one's natural care
Easter comes with joy and fun
And lots of chocolate for everyone
Read packet labels on your treats
So you'll be eating healthy sweets.

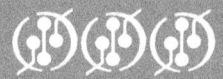

Certain months will bring a change
From hot to cold and wind to rain
We cherish the sun and the bright blue sea
And rug for the winter and snow that will be
We know that the year is passing so fast
And though winter's coming, it too shall not last
But, May holds a special celebration
For the person who shared in our tribulations
She gave comfort to us, offered words of praise
Happy Mother's Day, Mum, in my heart you will stay.

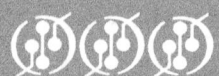

Christmas Holidays comes once a year
It is a time of Love and good Cheer
To all and everyone we need to say
Thank you to all and to all a good Day
Remember that happiness is always a choice
And you need to say it with a very strong voice
Look in the mirror and the person you see
Say loudly "There's no-one as special like Me"
Cry when you need and speak openly too
Cherish the body and spirit that's You
Everyone lives with a reason to be
So open your heart and let it fly free.

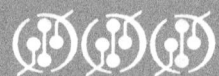

When we have these hot, humid days
We may go to swim and outside to play
Yet in the house the mould is flourishing
The places damp and wet are nourishing
Some types of growth can't be wiped away
And others in the walls will flourish and stay
You may not see as they grow in size
Yet their spores will travel and hurt your eyes
They may cause stomach upset, headaches & pain
You may just not be able to find strength again
Moisture and damp is its habitat
And the cleanest home can have mould impact.

Peta Zafir Publishing
www.petazafir.com
Peta Zafir You Tube Channel

BOOKS BY PETA ZAFIR
Health in Poetry Book 1
Health in Poetry Book 2
Book of Sayings Book 1
Book of Sayings Book 2
Book of Sayings Book 3
Book of Sayings Book 4
Scenar For Beginners

All books are available in print and eBook format from:
www.petazafir.com/books

Notes

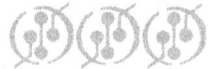

Your Poetry

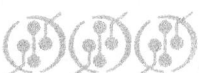

Notes

Your Poetry

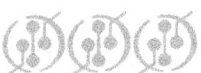

Notes

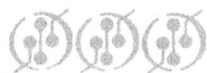

Your Poetry

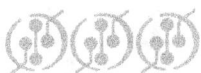

Notes

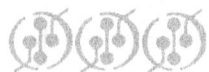

Your Poetry

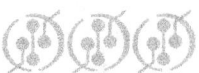

NOTES

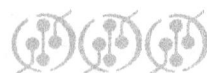

Your Poetry

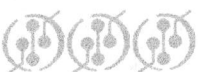

NOTES

Your Poetry

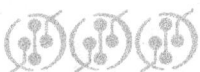

NOTES

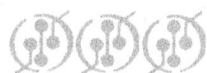

Your Poetry

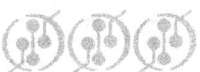

Notes

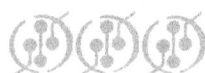

Your Poetry

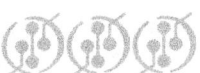

Notes

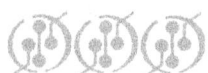

YOUR POETRY

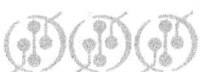

NOTES

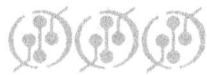

www.ingramcontent.com/pod-product-compliance
Lightning Source LLC
Chambersburg PA
CBHW071837290426
44109CB00017B/1837